DECODING LONGEVITY

Investigating the Intersection of Science, Art, and Culture in the Pursuit of a Longer Life.

By

Ruben M. McDonald

TABLE OF CONTENTS

INTRODUCTION

THE VALUE OF LONGEVITY IN CONTEMPORARY SOCIETY

The pursuit of longevity has drawn the interest of people and communities all around the world in an era marked by astounding advances in science and medicine. From prehistoric times, humans have had a basic drive to extend and improve the quality of life, which has shaped both scientific research and cultural norms. The book "Decoding Longevity: Investigating the Intersection of Science, Art, and

Culture in the Pursuit of a Longer Life."

" explores the complex relationship between science, art, and culture as it relates to our understanding of longevity and quest for a longer, healthier life.

In today's world, longevity—which is commonly interpreted as a longer life expectancy or the capacity to fend off the ravages of aging—is highly valued. Over the past century, human lifespans have increased dramatically due to breakthroughs in healthcare, diet, and technology. But the pursuit of long life goes beyond simply adding years to one's life; it also involves a comprehensive strategy for aging that prioritizes not only longevity but also vitality, quality of life, and overall well-being as one age.

To understand the origins of longevity practices and beliefs in ancient societies and civilizations, this investigation starts by looking at historical perspectives on longevity. Our knowledge of aging and longevity has developed throughout the ages of human experience and observation, from the search for immortality elixirs to the wisdom of longevity passed down through generations.

The biological underpinnings of longevity, which reveal the complex mechanisms of aging at the genetic, cellular, and molecular levels, are the central focus of the discussion. Developments in the fields of regenerative medicine, genetics, and epigenetics have opened new perspectives on the mechanisms underlying aging and age-related illnesses, perhaps leading to longer lifespans.

Further included in this investigation is the relationship between lifestyle factors and longevity, including the effects of nutrition and exercise as well as the significance of social support and mental health. Social conventions, behaviors, and attitudes about aging populations are greatly influenced by cultural conceptions of lifespan and aging.

As we learn more about the science of longevity, moral questions about the pursuit of extreme life extension and the effects of longer lifespans on society start to surface. Exploring visual depictions of aging, cultural differences in attitudes toward longevity, and the role of storytelling in imagining futures altered by longevity all contribute to an increasingly fascinating convergence of science, art, and culture.

Prospectively, the terrain of longevity is characterized by opportunities as well as difficulties. As aging and longevity continue to be redefined by new technology, ongoing study, and shifting social norms, significant concerns regarding equality, ethics, and what it means to live a longer life are brought to light.

To shed light on the complexity and opportunities surrounding the extension and enhancement of the human lifespan, "Decoding Longevity" encourages readers to join it on a voyage of discovery where science, art, and culture come together.

THE VALUE OF LONGEVITY IN CONTEMPORARY SOCIETY

In contemporary culture, the idea of longevity is extremely important since it reflects not just scientific advancements but also societal ideals, economic dynamics, and cultural goals. The comprehension of the consequences and prospects brought about by extended life is becoming more and more crucial as long life continues to rise in the world.

The global demographic changes that are taking place make lifespan one of the most important factors. A characteristic of many cultures is the aging population, as an increasing proportion of people live longer lives. The workforce, intergenerational relationships, retirement plans, and healthcare systems are all significantly impacted by this demographic shift. The goal of longevity research and policy activities is to solve the critical challenge of understanding how to assist and increase the well-being of aging populations while maintaining sustainable societal structures. Longevity offers advantages and disadvantages from an economic standpoint. On the one hand, a youthful, healthy aging population can greatly boost creativity, entrepreneurship, and economic production. The ideas, knowledge, and talents that older persons contribute to the workforce are invaluable, and creating conditions that encourage their ongoing involvement can have a positive economic impact. Conversely, the escalating expenses linked to age-related illnesses and long-term care pose financial difficulties that necessitate tactical planning and allocation of resources towards healthcare systems and social support networks.

Longevity also has an impact on ideas of well-being and quality of life. Living longer provides the opportunity for people to pursue meaningful experiences, continue learning throughout their lives, and stay involved in their communities well into old age. Yet, to guarantee that these prolonged years are marked by health, vigor, and social interaction, comprehensive strategies are needed, addressing not just medical interventions but also social determinants of health such as social support, education, and access to healthy settings.

In terms of culture, longevity affects the stories that are told about aging and elder adulthood as well as societal norms and values. Social views toward older persons are changing as a result of a shift in the perception of aging from one of decline to one of continuous development, learning, and contribution. These tales emphasize the relationship between art, culture, and the aging process and are shaped by artistic expressions, literature, media portrayals, and cultural behaviors. Research on longevity in science and technology is a promising area that could lead to discoveries in our understanding of the basic processes of aging, the creation of interventions to postpone age-related decline, and eventually, an extension of a healthy lifetime. This scientific project affects not just the health of the person but also larger societal issues, such as healthcare regulations, moral dilemmas, and public discussions about aging and long life.

To sum up, the value of longevity in contemporary society goes beyond simply counting the years. It takes into account factors that interact and influence how we view and experience aging, including demographic,

18 | P a g e

economic, social, cultural, and scientific aspects. The goal of "Decoding Longevity" is to examine these complicated aspects while acknowledging the potential and challenges that come with trying to live a longer, healthier, and more meaningful life.

HISTORICAL VIEWS OF LONGEVITY

Longevity is an enduring goal that has captured people's attention for ages; it is not a recent phenomenon. Views from the past regarding longevity paint a picture of the various cultural narratives, customs, and beliefs that surround the pursuit of immortality and the wish for longer life spans.

Many ancient societies had different ideas about how long people should live, and they frequently combined ideas about life, death, and the afterlife with their religious and cultural practices. For instance, the pursuit of immortality played a major role in religious rites and practices in ancient Egypt, where the afterlife journey and the preservation of life essence were emphasized in writings like the Book of the Dead and rituals related to graves. The study of longevity was also pursued by ancient Chinese societies, who employed methods including Taoist alchemy, herbal remedies, and longevity rituals to either achieve physical or spiritual immortality. These beliefs formed the basis of traditional Chinese medicine and longevity practices that persist to this day. The concept of "elixirs of life" and the quest for harmony with nature were central to these beliefs.

Stories of immortal gods and heroes such as Zeus, Hera, and Hercules expressed the desire for divine immortality and endless life in Greek and Roman mythology. Throughout history, explorers and adventurers have been captivated by the hunt for the fabled Fountain of Vigor, a fabled fountain that is said to grant longevity and vigor.

Alchemical experiments, herbal treatments, and the search for alchemical elixirs believed to grant immortality spurred a rebirth of interest in longevity in medieval and Renaissance Europe. The mysteries surrounding life extension and the quest for eternal youth were explored in the writings of philosophers like Roger Bacon and alchemists like Paracelsus. Lifespan was widely correlated with morality, wisdom, and spiritual enlightenment across all cultures and eras. The cultural tradition of longevity as a sign of honor and respect was influenced by the veneration of long-lived people as sages, seers, and keepers of ancient wisdom.

The study of aging and longevity moved from magical and alchemical domains to empirical research as scientific knowledge increased. The nature of life, aging, and the possibility of increasing human longevity through scientific discovery and technological advancement were among the topics of discussion among early modern philosophers like Leonardo da Vinci and Francis Bacon.

The historical viewpoints on longevity, which stretch from prehistoric times to the present, show a persistent human interest in prolonging life, being immortal, and pursuing everlasting vigor. These historical foundations still influence conversations and investigations into aging, longevity, and the science of prolonging a healthy lifespan in the modern era.

 Our book, "Decoding Longevity," delves into these historical accounts and charts the development of cultural conceptions, behaviors, and beliefs related to longevity while recognizing the persistent human desire to live longer, better lives, and find greater purpose in life.

CHAPTER 1

LONGEVITY PRACTICES AND ANCIENT CULTURES

The goal of discovering the keys to longevity and maintaining health and vitality throughout life was of great importance to ancient civilizations everywhere. They frequently combined their views on longevity techniques with their spiritual convictions, cultural customs, and firsthand observations of the natural world.

Ancient Egypt: Rituals and Elixirs

Longevity in ancient Egypt was intimately associated with belief systems surrounding the afterlife and religion. Because they thought that maintaining the physical body was crucial to a smooth transition to the afterlife, the Egyptians employed complex mummification techniques. Additionally, thought to bestow vitality and ward off aging were elixirs and potions derived from herbs, minerals, and animal parts. Remedies and prescriptions for treating age-related ailments and promoting longevity can be found in the Ebers Papyrus, one of the oldest medical texts.

Traditional Chinese Medicine and Taoist Knowledge

Chinese culture has a long history of using herbal remedies and Taoist philosophy to promote longevity. In their search for the secret of immortality, Taoist alchemists blended the study of qi (life energy) with herbal remedies, breath work, and meditation. Traditional Chinese medicine (TCM) prescribes herbal tonics, acupuncture, and qigong exercises to promote longevity and well-being. TCM places a strong emphasis on balance, harmony, and preventive care.

Philosophical Considerations on Classical Greece and Rome

The nature of life, aging, and longevity were topics of discussion for philosophers and scholars in ancient Greece and Rome. The Stoics promoted virtue, moderation, and philosophical reflection as means of achieving a happy and meaningful life. These philosophers included Seneca and Marcus Aurelius. Greek doctors like Hippocrates stressed the value of environmental variables, physical activity, and diet in preserving health and extending life.

Indigenous Nations: Knowledge Derived from Nature

Indigenous peoples have long been familiar with the subtle uses of indigenous plants, herbs, and natural treatments to enhance health and prolong life. They believed that a holistic approach to well-being included practices like herbal medicine, shamanic healing, and ceremonial ceremonies. Generation after generation of traditional wisdom-guided behaviors meant to promote health and longevity by emphasizing the interdependence of people, the natural world, and the spiritual realm. Ancient Indian Wisdom, or Ayurveda The full framework for promoting lifespan and holistic health is provided by India's traditional medical system, Ayurveda. Ayurvedic treatments include herbal remedies, detoxification therapies, yoga, meditation, and nutritional advice. They are based on the theories of doshas (body-mind kinds) and the equilibrium of prana (life force). Comprehensive guidelines on longevity-promoting techniques that are specific to each person's constitution and imbalances can be found in Ayurvedic literature such as the Sushruta Samhita and Charaka Samhita.

Native American Customs: American Wisdom

Different approaches to lifespan and health maintenance were created by indigenous cultures in the Americas,

including the Maya, Aztecs, and other
Native American tribes. Key
components of their wellness approach
included herbal medicine, sweat lodges,
healing ceremonies, and customary
food and lifestyle choices. As guardians
of wisdom, elders were highly
esteemed in their cultures for imparting
knowledge and customs that bolstered
resiliency, vibrancy, and longevity.

An understanding of ancient societies'
longevity customs reveals a deep
reverence for the interdependence of
the mind, body, spirit, and
environment. The fundamental ideas of

harmony, balance, and holistic well-being are still relevant in contemporary approaches to longevity and health promotion, even though particular methods and ideologies differ greatly.

IMPORTANT ASPECTS OF RESEARCH ON LONGEVITY

Significant advancements in the field of longevity study have resulted from science's ongoing focus on understanding and extending human lifespan. These milestones reflect major developments, discoveries, and paradigm shifts that have changed our understanding of aging, health span, and the factors that influence lifespan.

In the 1980s, Telomerase and Telomeres were discovered.

When Elizabeth Blackburn, Carol Greider, and Jack Szostak discovered telomeres and telomerase in the 1980s, it was one of the turning points in the study of longevity. Cell replication and aging are significantly influenced by telomeres, the protective caps at the ends of chromosomes. The telomerase enzyme, which keeps the telomeres long, has emerged as a key player in the knowledge of cellular senescence and the possibility of telomere-based therapies for disorders associated with aging.

Investigations of Caloric Restriction (1930s to Present)

Studying calorie restriction—a technique that lowers intake without causing malnutrition—has provided important new information about the processes underlying aging and long life. Research on a variety of species, such as rodents and primates, has demonstrated that calorie restriction can improve metabolic health, postpone age-related illnesses, and increase lifespan. Research on metabolic regulation, nutrient-sensing pathways, and the impact of dietary changes on longevity have all been sparked by these discoveries.

Finding the Longevity Genes (1990s–Present)

Thanks to developments in genetics and genomics, genes and pathways linked to longevity have been found. Genes like SIRT1, FOXO, and mTOR that are important in controlling aging processes, cellular stress responses, and lifespan extension have been found through studies in model species including C. elegans, fruit flies, and mice. The comprehension of the genetic foundation for extended lifespan has created opportunities for focused therapies and medication creation aimed at age-related processes.

Neuroprotective Substances and Measures

Research on longevity has accelerated the investigation of neuroprotective substances and therapies. Preclinical research has demonstrated the potential for compounds like rapamycin, metformin, resveratrol (found in red wine), and NAD+ precursors to improve health span and lengthen lifespan. To validate the safety and effectiveness of these interventions in humans and to develop new anti-aging medications, clinical trials, and ongoing research are being conducted.

From the 2010s to the Present, Senolytics and Senescence Clearance Age-related disorders and aging are associated with senescence; an irreversible cell cycle stop condition. Senolytics are substances that target and eradicate senescent cells specifically, encouraging tissue regeneration and postponing the deterioration that comes with aging. With potential applications in the treatment of age-related diseases such as osteoarthritis, cardiovascular disease, and dementia, the development of senolytic treatments and senescence clearance technologies provides a promising direction in longevity research.

Multiomic Approaches and Systems Biology

The study of lifespan has been transformed by developments in computer modeling, systems biology, and omics technologies (genomics, transcriptomics, proteomics, and metabolomics). These integrated approaches allow for detailed examination of aging-related processes, identification of aging biomarkers, and customized therapies based on unique health profiles. To achieve longer lifespans and improved health, data science, technology, and healthcare are coming together to create individualized longevity strategies and precision medicine.

 Studies on Human Longevity and Non-Human Primates

Nonhuman primate longitudinal studies, like the current work at the National Institute on Aging's

Nonhuman Primate Aging and Caloric Restriction Database, offer important new information about the course of aging, health outcomes, and longevity-influencing therapies. Our understanding of the genetic, environmental, and lifestyle factors that lead to long and healthy lives is aided by studies on human longevity, such as population-based research, genetic cohort analysis, and centenarian studies.

These landmarks in the field of longevity study highlight the multidisciplinary character of aging science, which includes systems biology, genetics, cellular biology, metabolism, epigenetics, and translational medicine. The worldwide community of researchers, doctors, and innovators is making significant strides in deciphering the mysteries of longevity and enhancing the health of aging populations.

THE BIOLOGICAL BASIS OF LIFESPAN

A complex interaction of genetic, cellular, molecular, and environmental factors affects longevity, or the capacity to live a long and healthy life. To decipher the mechanisms of aging, locate viable therapies, and encourage healthy aging throughout the lifespan, it is imperative to comprehend the biological underpinnings of longevity.

Genetics and Lifespan

A person's longevity is mostly determined by their genetics. Genes involved in DNA repair, cellular maintenance, immunological function, and metabolism are among the genetic variations linked to longer lifespans that have been found via studies of centenarians and long-lived societies.

Although longevity estimates' heritability varies throughout populations, they usually point to a genetic component to lifespan variation.

Age-Related Cellular Mechanisms

Aging is defined as a progressive loss of homeostasis and cellular function at the cellular level. Important biological pathways linked to aging comprise: With every cell division, the protective caps known as telomeres that are located at the ends of chromosomes shorten. Cellular senescence and age-related illnesses are linked to telomere attrition.

Mitochondrial Dysfunction: As we age, our cells' energy-producing powerhouses, the mitochondria, experience a functional decline and damage accumulation. Oxidative stress, inflammation, and cellular aging are all influenced by mitochondrial malfunction.

Senescent cells that stop dividing but have metabolic activity over time build up in tissues called cellular senescence.

Senescent cells contribute to tissue dysfunction and age-related diseases by secreting chemicals that promote inflammation.

Alterations in Epigenetics: Aging-related changes in non-coding RNA regulation, histone modifications, and DNA methylation are examples of epigenetic modifications that affect gene expression patterns. Changes in epigenetic markers have the potential to affect cellular processes and give rise to age-related characteristics.

How Epigenetics Affects Longevity

To control the aging process, epigenetics—the study of heritable variations in gene expression without changes to the underlying DNA sequence—is essential. Environmental influences, lifestyle decisions, and developmental cues can all have an impact on epigenetic alterations. Age-associated DNA methylation patterns serve as the basis for epigenetic clocks, biomarkers that have been created to estimate lifespan and measure biological age.

Environmental and Lifestyle Elements

Longevity is influenced by environmental and lifestyle variables in addition to genetics and biological mechanisms. Nutrition: A balanced diet high in vitamins, minerals, antioxidants, and phytonutrients supports cellular health and resilience, which in turn promotes healthy aging.

Physical Activity: Longevity is enhanced by regular exercise, which also increases muscle strength, mobility, cardiovascular health, and cognitive function.

Stress management: Inflammation and chronic stress hasten the aging process. Stress-reduction techniques that increase resilience and well-being include mindfulness, meditation, and social support.

The quality of sleep is crucial for immune system function, cellular repair, cognitive function, and general wellness.

Avoiding Hazardous Substances: Reducing exposure to smoke, excessive drinking, chemicals found in the environment, and UV radiation from the sun promotes good aging and longevity.

Regenerative Medicine and Longevity

Improvements in tissue engineering, stem cell therapies, regenerative medicine, and regenerative interventions have the potential to lengthen healthy lifespans. In longevity science, research is currently being conducted on methods to improve tissue repair, restore damaged organs, and revitalize cellular function.

53 | P a g e

It takes an integrated approach integrating genetics, cellular biology, epigenetics, environmental impacts, and lifestyle factors to understand the scientific underpinnings of longevity. Researchers seek to create interventions that increase the quality of life and longevity across the lifespan by clarifying the mechanics of aging and discovering modifiable factors that promote healthy aging.

CHAPTER 2

THE STUDY OF GENETICS AND ITS RELATIONSHIP TO LIFESPAN.

The influence of genetics on lifespan has been the focus of much scientific investigation. Although lifestyle, environmental conditions, and chance occurrences have a considerable impact on longevity, genetic characteristics also have a substantial influence on an individual's potential for a long and healthy life.

Genes and variants associated with longevity

Research on centenarians, persons who reach the age of 100 or more, has identified distinct genetic variations linked to longer lifespans. These genes that are connected with longevity frequently affect important biological processes that contribute to the duration of good health and lifespan. Examples of such genes include:

Variants in the APOE gene are linked to both the risk of developing Alzheimer's disease and the potential for living a longer life. The APOE ε4 variation is connected to an increased risk of Alzheimer's but decreased risk of cardiovascular disease in some groups.

The FOXO3 gene plays a role in controlling cellular stress responses, DNA repair, and insulin signaling. Variants in FOXO3 have been related to remarkable lifespans in numerous populations, including centenarians.

SIRT1: SIRT1 is a gene implicated in cellular metabolism, stress response, and longevity pathways. Activation of SIRT1 has been associated with lifespan extension in animal studies, while its implications in humans are currently under investigation.

MTOR: The MTOR gene has a function in nutrition sensing, cellular growth, and metabolism. Genetic polymorphisms in MTOR have been connected with lifespan and age-related illnesses, underlining its role in aging processes.

KLOTHO: The KLOTHO gene encodes a protein that controls aging-related pathways, including insulin signaling and oxidative stress response. Variants in KLOTHO have been associated with longevity and cognitive performance in humans.

HERITABILITY OF LONGEVITY

The heritability of longevity refers to the extent to which hereditary variables contribute to variations in lifespan within a group. Studies of familial longevity, where numerous members of a family display outstanding lifespan, have revealed insights into the genetic foundation of longevity. Twin studies have also proven a genetic component to lifespan variance, with estimates of heritability ranging from roughly 20% to 30% to as high as 50% in some groups.

Genetic Influences on Aging Processes

Genetic factors influence aging processes at numerous levels, from cellular mechanisms to systemic pathways that determine overall health span. Key areas where genetics play a role in aging include:

DNA Repair Mechanisms: Genes involved in DNA repair, such as those in the nucleotide excision repair and base excision repair pathways, assist in maintaining genomic stability and defend against age-related DNA damage.

Inflammatory Response: Genetic differences in immune-related genes can alter inflammatory responses and immunological function, affecting susceptibility to age-related inflammation and chronic illnesses.

 Metabolic Regulation: Genes involved in metabolism, energy balance, and mitochondrial function control cellular metabolism and energy generation, which in turn affect aging processes and longevity.

Polygenic Influences on Longevity

Longevity is a complex feature impacted by several hereditary factors, each contributing a minor effect on overall lifetime. Polygenic scores, determined based on the cumulative impact of several genetic variants related to longevity, can provide insights into an individual's genetic predisposition for longevity. Polygenic risk scores are used in research to evaluate the cumulative influence of genetic polymorphisms on lifespan and age-related variables.

Genetic Testing and Longevity Prediction

Advances in genomic technologies, including as whole-genome sequencing and genome-wide association studies (GWAS), have allowed the identification of genetic variations associated with longevity. While genetic testing can provide information on individual genetic risk factors and predispositions, it's crucial to recognize that genetics is just one aspect of the complex interplay between genes, environment, and lifestyle in determining health span and lifespan. In conclusion, genetics plays a substantial role in affecting longevity, with certain genes and genetic variations implicated in age-related processes, illness vulnerability, and lifespan variance. Understanding the genetic basis of longevity contributes to our knowledge of aging mechanisms, personalized medicine methods, and therapies targeted at promoting healthy aging and prolonging lifespan.

Cellular Mechanisms of Aging

Aging is a complex biological process marked by a steady deterioration in cellular function and tissue integrity. Understanding the biological mechanics of aging is vital for deciphering the underlying causes of age-related disorders and devising therapies to promote healthy aging.

Telomere Shortening and Cellular Senescence

Telomeres are protective caps at the ends of chromosomes that shorten with each cell cycle. Telomere shortening is considered a hallmark of aging, as critically short telomeres promote cellular senescence—a state of irreversible cell cycle stop. Senescent cells develop with aging and contribute to tissue malfunction and inflammation. Telomere maintenance mechanisms, including the enzyme telomerase, play a role in controlling cellular lifetime and senescence.

Mitochondrial Dysfunction and Oxidative Stress

Mitochondria, the energy-producing organelles in cells, are crucial to cellular metabolism and play a role in aging processes. Mitochondrial dysfunction, defined by reduced energy generation, increased reactive oxygen species (ROS) production, and impaired mitochondrial quality control, is associated with aging and age-related illnesses. Oxidative stress resulting from ROS accumulation can harm cellular components and contribute to cellular aging and degeneration.

DNA Damage and Repair

Accumulation of DNA damage over time is a fundamental component of aging. Endogenous factors such as ROS, environmental exposures, and metabolic activities can produce DNA damage. Cells contain mechanisms for repairing DNA damage, including base excision repair, nucleotide excision repair, and double-strand break repair pathways. However, with age, DNA repair efficiency may drop, leading to genomic instability and increased vulnerability to age-related illnesses.

Cellular Senescence and Inflammation

Senescent cells, while no longer proliferating, remain metabolically active and release pro-inflammatory chemicals, a condition known as the senescence-associated secretory phenotype (SASP). SASP components contribute to chronic low-grade inflammation, or inflammation, which is implicated in age-related diseases such as cardiovascular disease, neurodegeneration, and cancer. Targeting senescent cells and inflammation is a focus of anti-aging research.

Epigenetic Changes

Epigenetic alterations, such as DNA methylation, histone modifications, and non-coding RNA regulation, influence gene expression patterns without altering the underlying DNA sequence. Age-related epigenetic alterations can impact cellular function, gene expression profiles, and cellular identity. Epigenetic clocks, based on age-associated epigenetic markers, provide insights into biological aging and can forecast chronological age and health span.

Proteostasis and Cellular Quality Control

Proteostasis refers to the maintenance of protein homeostasis within cells, including protein production, folding, and destruction. Age-related deterioration in proteostasis can lead to protein misfolding, aggregation, and buildup of damaged proteins. Cellular quality control mechanisms, such as chaperones, autophagy, and the ubiquitin-proteasome system, assist in maintaining protein integrity and avoid cellular damage associated with aging.

Stem Cell Exhaustion and Tissue Regeneration

Stem cells perform a critical function in tissue regeneration and repair throughout life. With aging, stem cell populations may drop in quantity and function, leading to lower tissue regeneration potential and compromised repair processes. Stem cell exhaustion contributes to age-related reduction in organ function and regeneration capacity.

Understanding the complicated biological mechanisms of aging is crucial to creating therapies that address underlying causes of age-related disorders, promote healthy aging, and increase health span. Strategies focused on preserving cellular integrity, increasing repair mechanisms, and altering age-related pathways hold promise for tackling the issues of an aging population and improving quality of life in later years.

ROLE OF EPIGENETICS IN LONGEVITY

Epigenetics, the study of heritable changes in gene expression that do not entail mutations to the DNA sequence itself, plays a vital role in controlling aging processes and impacting lifespan. Epigenetic alterations can impact gene activity, cellular function, and organismal health, contributing to the complex interplay between genetics, environment, and lifestyle variables in determining lifespan.

DNA Methylation and Age-Associated Changes

DNA methylation, the addition of methyl groups to DNA molecules, is a significant epigenetic alteration that undergoes age-associated modifications. Global DNA methylation patterns can fluctuate with age, resulting in modifications in gene expression profiles and cellular function. DNA methylation clocks, based on age-related methylation changes at specific CpG sites, are used to measure biological age and forecast lifespan.

Histone Modifications and Chromatin Structure

Histone changes, such as acetylation, methylation, and phosphorylation, alter chromatin shape and gene accessibility.

Changes in histone marks during aging can impact gene expression patterns, cellular senescence, and epigenetic regulation. Histone deacetylase inhibitors and histone methyl transferase inhibitors are being studied as potential therapies to control aging-related epigenetic alterations.

Non-Coding RNAs and Regulatory Networks

Non-coding RNAs, including microRNAs (miRNAs) and long non-coding RNAs (lncRNAs), perform roles in post-transcriptional gene regulation and epigenetic modification. MiRNAs can target mRNAs for destruction or translational repression, impacting cellular processes associated with aging and longevity. LncRNAs function in chromatin remodeling, transcriptional control, and cellular senescence pathways.

Epigenetic Clocks and Biological Age

Epigenetic clocks, based on age-related epigenetic alterations, provide insights into biological age and health span. Methylation-based clocks, such as the Horvath clock and the Hannum clock, correlate with chronological age but also represent age-related changes in cellular function, illness risk, and mortality. Epigenetic age acceleration, assessed by deviations from chronological age, has been associated with age-related disorders and death outcomes.

Environmental Influences on Epigenetics

Environmental factors, including nutrition, exercise, stress, pollution, and lifestyle choices, can alter epigenetic patterns and modify gene expression profiles. Nutritional therapies, such as calorie restriction and dietary supplementation with bioactive chemicals, can alter epigenetic control of aging-related pathways. Epigenetic responses to environmental cues contribute to individual diversity in aging trajectories and illness vulnerability.

Epigenetic Regulation of Longevity Pathways

Epigenetic alterations affect important longevity processes, including those involved in cellular senescence, DNA repair, oxidative stress response, and metabolic regulation. Epigenetic control of genes related to aging, such as FOXO3, SIRT1, and KLOTHO, modifies longevity and health span in model organisms and human populations. Targeting epigenetic regulators and pathways shows promise for therapies targeted at promoting healthy aging and increasing longevity.

Epigenetic Drift and Aging Phenotypes

Epigenetic drift, characterized by random variations in DNA methylation and chromatin modifications across time, leads to age-related epigenetic alterations and heterogeneity among people. Epigenetic signatures associated with aging phenotypes, disease risk, and physiological changes can serve as biomarkers for monitoring health span, forecasting outcomes, and assessing therapies aiming at slowing down or reversing age-related epigenetic changes.

Understanding the function of epigenetics in longevity provides insights into the biological mechanics of aging, disease vulnerability, and individual variability in aging trajectories. Epigenetic therapies, including epigenetic modifiers, lifestyle modifications, and tailored techniques, offer prospective pathways for promoting healthy aging, postponing age-related disorders, and boosting the quality of life in aging populations.

SCIENTIFIC APPROACHES TO PROLONGING LIFE

Advancements in science and medicine have led to creative treatments aimed at prolonging life and boosting health span, the time of life free from major disease and impairment. These scientific techniques comprise a spectrum of strategies targeting biological, cellular, and environmental aspects to promote healthy aging and lengthen lifespan.

Genetic Interventions

Longevity Genes: Research on longevity-associated genes, such as FOXO3, SIRT1, and KLOTHO, has stimulated interest in genetic therapies to modulate aging processes. Gene editing technologies, such as CRISPR-

Cas9, show potential for targeted changes to boost lifespan pathways and prevent age-related decline.

Telomere Maintenance: Strategies to maintain telomere length and telomerase activity, such as telomerase activation therapies and telomere-targeted gene therapies, are under investigation for their potential to delay cellular senescence and promote healthy aging.

Pharmacological Interventions

Senolytics: Senolytic medications target and destroy senescent cells, which grow with aging and lead to tissue malfunction and inflammation. Senolytics, such as dasatinib and quercetin, have shown promise in preclinical research for renewing tissues and increasing health span.

Metabolic Modulators: Compounds that target metabolic pathways, such as rapamycin (mTOR inhibitor), metformin (AMPK activator), and resveratrol (SIRT1 activator), are being explored for their potential to promote cellular resilience, postpone aging processes, and improve overall health.

Regenerative Medicine

Stem Cell Therapies: Stem cell-based techniques for tissue regeneration and repair hold promise for tackling age-related degenerative disorders, such as osteoarthritis, cardiovascular disease, and dementia. Induced pluripotent stem cells (iPSCs) and tissue engineering approaches are boosting regenerative medicine applications.

Organ Regeneration: Research into organ regeneration, including bioengineered organs, organoids, and tissue scaffolds, aims to restore organ function and improve the quality of life for aging populations. Strategies for increasing organ repair processes and fostering tissue regeneration are areas of active inquiry.

Nutritional and Lifestyle Interventions

Caloric Restriction: Caloric restriction, without malnutrition, has been demonstrated to prolong longevity and improve health span in numerous creatures. Research continues to examine the processes underpinning caloric restriction's effects on metabolism, cellular signaling, and lifespan pathways.

Nutritional Supplements

Nutraceuticals and dietary supplements, such as antioxidants, polyphenols, omega-3 fatty acids, and micronutrients, are explored for their potential to maintain cellular health, reduce oxidative stress, and modify aging-related pathways.

Physical Activity: Regular exercise, including aerobic, resistance, and high-intensity training, has dramatic impacts on cardiovascular health, muscle strength, cognitive function, and overall well-being. Exercise interventions for elderly people attempt to maintain physical function, mobility, and independence.

Anti-inflammatory and Anti-Aging Therapies

Anti-Inflammatory Agents: Chronic inflammation is a hallmark of aging and age-related illnesses. Anti-inflammatory medicines, dietary anti-inflammatory substances, and lifestyle therapies target inflammatory pathways to reduce inflammation and improve health outcomes.

Anti-Aging Skin Therapies: Advances in dermatology and cosmeceuticals have led to the creation of anti-aging skin therapies, such as topical antioxidants, retinoids, peptides, and growth factors, to battle skin aging and promote skin health.

Personalized Medicine Approaches

Precision Aging: Personalized medical approaches, including genomics, epigenetics, biomarkers, and digital health technology, offer precision aging strategies tailored to individual health profiles, genetic susceptibilities, and lifestyle factors.

Health Monitoring: Wearable gadgets, digital health platforms, and artificial intelligence applications offer real-time health monitoring, early disease detection, and individualized therapies for optimizing health span and lifespan.

The convergence of these scientific techniques, coupled with current research in aging biology, systems biology, and translational medicine, shows promise for prolonging healthy lifespan, preventing age-related disorders, and boosting quality of life in aging populations. Multidisciplinary collaboration among researchers, clinicians, politicians, and industry stakeholders is vital for converting scientific discoveries into effective interventions for improving lifespan and well-being.

CHAPTER 3

ANTI-AGING THERAPIES: MYTHS VS. FACTS

Myth: Anti-aging medications may reverse the aging process. Fact: While some anti-aging therapies can slow down specific parts of aging and enhance overall health, they cannot reverse the aging process. Aging is a complicated biological phenomenon impacted by genetic, environmental, and lifestyle variables.

 Myth: Anti-aging products can remove wrinkles and restore youthful skin overnight. Fact: Anti-aging creams and skincare products can enhance skin texture, hydration, and look over time with constant use. However, they cannot remove wrinkles or turn back the clock on aging skin. Results vary depending on individual skin types and the substances utilized in the products. Myth: Hormone replacement treatment (HRT) is a one-size-fits-all answer for anti-aging. Fact: Hormone replacement therapy, such as estrogen or testosterone replacement, may be advantageous for some persons experiencing hormonal abnormalities associated with aging. However, HRT is not good for everyone, and its dangers and benefits should be carefully reviewed by healthcare specialists based on individual health profiles and medical history.

Myth: Supplements and vitamins can cure aging and prolong lives. Fact: While nutritional supplements and vitamins have a role in maintaining overall health and well-being, no miracle pill can reverse aging or lengthen lifespan on its own. A balanced diet, frequent exercise, proper sleep, and good living behaviors are critical components of optimal aging.

Myth: Cosmetic procedures like Botox and fillers are the only effective anti-aging therapies. Fact: Cosmetic procedures like Botox injections and dermal fillers can address specific indicators of aging, such as wrinkles and volume loss. However, these are not the only effective anti-aging therapy. Non-invasive procedures, skincare routines, lifestyle alterations, and preventative healthcare measures also play essential roles in anti-aging efforts.

Myth: Anti-aging medicines are only for older folks. Fact: Anti-aging therapies, including skincare, nutrition, exercise, and stress management, are good for individuals of all ages. Prevention and early intervention are fundamental ideas in anti-aging strategies, helping to maintain health, energy, and quality of life over the lifespan.

Myth: All-natural or organic products are always safe and effective for anti-aging. Fact: While natural and organic skincare products may offer benefits such as less exposure to synthetic chemicals, not all natural components are safe or effective for anti-aging purposes. It's crucial to examine elements such as formulation, ingredient quality, scientific proof, and individual skin sensitivity when choosing anti-aging solutions.

Myth: Anti-aging methods involve pricey treatments or surgeries. Fact: Effective anti-aging measures don't usually require pricey treatments or surgeries. Simple lifestyle adjustments, such as a good diet, regular exercise, appropriate sleep, stress management, and sun protection, can have tremendous effects on aging healthily. Consultation with healthcare professionals can help adapt anti-aging techniques to specific requirements and finances.

In short, differentiating myths from realities about anti-aging therapy is vital for making informed decisions about health, skincare, and overall well-being. While there is no fountain of youth, taking a holistic approach to healthy aging can contribute to a vigorous and meaningful life at any age.

EMERGING TECHNOLOGIES IN LONGEVITY RESEARCH

Advancements in science and technology are generating creative methods to understanding aging processes, prolonging health span, and promoting longevity. Emerging technologies in longevity study involve several fields, from genetics and regenerative medicine to artificial intelligence and digital health, giving new insights and prospects for increasing human health and lifespan.

Genomics and Precision Medicine

Genome Sequencing: Next-generation sequencing technologies have transformed genomics research, enabling thorough investigation of genetic variants, epigenetic alterations, and gene expression profiles associated with aging and age-related disorders. Whole-genome sequencing, single-cell sequencing, and epigenomic profiling approaches provide insights into personalized aging trajectories and illness susceptibilities.

Precision Aging: Precision medicine approaches leverage genomic data, biomarkers, and digital health technologies to design individualized interventions for optimizing health span and preventing age-related illnesses. Precision aging projects focus on individualized risk assessment, early illness detection, targeted medicines, and lifestyle interventions matched to genetic profiles and health goals.

REGENERATIVE MEDICINE AND TISSUE ENGINEERING

Stem Cell Therapies: Advances in stem cell research, including induced pluripotent stem cells (iPSCs), adult stem cells, and tissue-specific progenitor cells, show promise for tissue regeneration, organ repair, and rejuvenation therapies. Stem cell-based treatments attempt to restore cellular function, promote tissue resilience, and mitigate age-related degenerative changes.

Organoids and 3D Bioprinting: Organoids, small organ models

produced from stem cells, provide platforms for researching organ development, disease modeling, and drug screening in personalized medicine. 3D bioprinting technologies enable the manufacture of bioengineered tissues and organs, presenting possible solutions for organ transplantation, regenerative medicines, and customized healthcare.

Artificial Intelligence and Data Analytics

Machine Learning: Machine learning algorithms evaluate large-scale omics data, electronic health records, imaging data, and clinical outcomes to detect trends, forecast disease trajectories, and optimize treatment methods. AI-driven methods for biomarker discovery, medication development, and patient stratification enhance precision medicine projects in aging research. Longevity Prediction Models: AI-powered longevity prediction models, based on multi-omic data, lifestyle factors, and environmental impacts, aim to estimate biological age, forecast lifetime, and assess health span trajectories. Longitudinal data analysis and deep learning algorithms boost understanding of aging mechanisms and individual heterogeneity in aging phenotypes.

Digital Health Technologies

Wearable Devices: Wearable sensors, fitness trackers, and health monitoring devices collect real-time data on physiological parameters, activity levels, sleep patterns, and vital signs. Integrating wearable technology with AI analytics offers continuous health monitoring, early symptom diagnosis, and personalized wellness interventions.

Telemedicine and Remote Monitoring: Telehealth platforms, remote monitoring systems, and virtual care services offer remote consultations, illness management, and healthcare delivery to elderly populations. Telemedicine technologies increase access to healthcare, promote patient participation, and support aging-in-place efforts.

Nutrigenomics and Metabolic Health

Nutrigenomics: Nutrigenomics explores the relationship between nutrition, genetics, and health outcomes, discovering dietary components that influence aging processes, metabolic pathways, and disease risk. Personalized nutrition interventions based on genetic profiles and metabolic characteristics optimize dietary strategies for healthy aging.

Metabolic Health Monitoring

Metabolic profiling technologies, such as metabolomics and lipidomics, examine metabolic biomarkers, metabolic pathways, and metabolic fingerprints linked with aging-related disorders. Metabolic health monitoring informs individualized therapies for metabolic syndrome, insulin resistance, mitochondrial dysfunction, and age-related metabolic diseases.

Emerging technologies in longevity research are revolutionizing our understanding of aging biology, disease pathways, and tailored healthcare.

Integrating multidisciplinary methods, data-driven insights, and new interventions supports collaborative efforts to extend health span, enhance quality of life, and promote successful aging for individuals and populations globally.

LONGEVITY AND REGENERATIVE MEDICINE

Regenerative medicine, a multidisciplinary area focusing on utilizing the body's natural repair mechanisms to restore tissue function and cure damaged organs, connects with longevity research in fundamental ways. By tackling cellular senescence, tissue regeneration, and age-related degenerative disorders, regenerative medicine shows promise for prolonging health span and increasing quality of life in aging populations.

Stem Cells and Tissue Regeneration

Stem Cell Therapies: Stem cells, with their unique ability to develop into numerous cell types and regenerate themselves, are crucial players in regenerative medicine. Adult stem cells, induced pluripotent stem cells (iPSCs), and tissue-specific progenitor cells offer options for tissue regeneration, organ repair, and rejuvenation therapy.

Tissue Engineering: Tissue engineering combines stem cells, biomaterials, and bioengineering techniques to build functional tissues and organs. Bioengineered tissues, such as skin grafts, cartilage implants, and organoids, show promise for tackling age-related degeneration, injury repair, and organ transplantation problems.

Reversing Cellular Senescence

Senolytics: Senolytic medications target and destroy senescent cells, which grow with age and contribute to tissue malfunction, inflammation, and age-related illnesses. Senolytics rejuvenate tissues, boost regenerative capacity, and attenuate age-related decline by eliminating senescent cells and facilitating tissue regeneration.

Senescence Clearance tactics: In addition to senolytics, senescence clearance tactics include immune-based therapy, genetic interventions, and senescent cell ablation procedures. By eliminating senescent cells and restoring tissue homeostasis, these techniques attempt to increase health span and delay age-related diseases.

Metabolic Health and Longevity

Metabolic Interventions: Metabolic health influences aging processes, cellular function, and regenerative ability. Nutritional therapies, caloric restriction mimetics, and metabolic modulators target metabolic pathways, energy metabolism, and nutrition-sensing mechanisms to improve longevity and boost tissue resilience.

Mitochondrial Function: Mitochondria, the cellular powerhouses responsible for energy production, play a critical role in aging and regenerative processes. Enhancing mitochondrial function, lowering oxidative stress, and increasing mitochondrial quality control systems improve cellular health, tissue repair, and lifespan.

Aging Biomarkers and Personalized Regenerative Therapies

Biomarker Discovery: Biomarkers of aging, such as epigenetic clocks, telomere length, inflammatory markers, and metabolic indicators, influence individualized regenerative therapies. Biomarker assessments guide treatment choices, monitor regeneration responses, and optimize therapies for aging-related disorders.

 Precision Medicine Approaches: Precision regenerative medicine incorporates genomic data, biomarker profiles, and patient-specific characteristics to adapt therapy to individual needs and health profiles. Precision medicine tactics enhance regenerative outcomes, limit risks, and improve patient outcomes in aging populations.

Regenerative Strategies for Age-Related Diseases

Neurodegeneration: Regenerative medicine techniques for neurodegenerative illnesses, such as Alzheimer's, Parkinson's, and age-related cognitive decline, focus on neuroprotection, neurogenesis stimulation, and neural circuit restoration. Stem cell therapies, neurotrophic factors, and brain-machine interfaces offer promising answers for age-related neurological diseases.

Cardiovascular Regeneration

Cardiovascular regenerative medicines target heart failure, vascular aging, and age-related cardiovascular disorders. Stem cell transplantation, cardiac tissue engineering, and regenerative cardiac patches attempt to restore heart function, improve vascular health, and extend cardiovascular health span.

In conclusion, the integration of regenerative medicine principles with longevity research gives prospects to address age-related issues, accelerate tissue regeneration, and promote healthy aging. By leveraging regenerative therapies, cellular rejuvenation techniques, and tailored interventions, regenerative medicine contributes to prolonging health span, increasing quality of life, and expanding the frontiers of longevity science.

Lifestyle Factors and Longevity

Lifestyle variables play a major influence in influencing lifespan and total health span—the time of life lived in excellent health without substantial disease or impairment. Adopting good living practices can prolong longevity, prevent age-related decline, and improve quality of life as persons' age.

Nutrition and Diet

Balanced Diet: Consuming a balanced diet rich in fruits, vegetables, whole grains, lean meats, and healthy fats delivers important nutrients, antioxidants, and phytochemicals that support cellular health and immunological function. Diets heavy in processed foods, carbohydrates, and saturated fats contribute to inflammation, oxidative stress, and chronic illnesses.

Caloric Intake: Caloric restriction, without malnutrition, has been associated with improved lifespan and health span in numerous creatures. Moderate calorie intake, portion control, and mindful eating behaviors promote metabolic health, weight management, and lifespan by reducing the risk of obesity, diabetes, and cardiovascular illnesses.

Physical Activity and Exercise

Regular Exercise: Engaging in regular physical activity, including aerobic exercise, strength training, flexibility exercises, and balance activities, enhances cardiovascular fitness, muscle strength, bone density, and cognitive function. Exercise also promotes mood, decreases stress, and improves overall well-being, contributing to good aging.

Daily exercise: Incorporating daily exercise, such as walking, cycling, gardening, or using the stairs, lowers sedentary behavior and promotes an active lifestyle. Maintaining mobility, joint flexibility, and functional independence through frequent activity increases longevity and reduces age-related loss in physical function.

Stress Management and Mental Well-Being

Stress Reduction: Chronic stress promotes aging processes, adds to inflammation, and affects immunological function. Stress management strategies, such as mindfulness meditation, deep breathing exercises, yoga, and relaxation therapies, build emotional resilience, reduce cortisol levels, and enhance coping mechanisms for stress.

Social Connections: Maintaining social connections, developing relationships, and engaging in social activities are crucial for mental well-being and longevity. Social support networks, meaningful connections, and community involvement promote a sense of belonging, purpose, and emotional support, buffering against loneliness and isolation.

Sleep Quality and Restorative Sleep

Sleep Hygiene: Prioritizing excellent sleep hygiene habits, such as maintaining a regular sleep schedule, providing a comfortable sleep environment, limiting screen time before bedtime, and avoiding coffee or heavy meals at night, improves sleep quality and promotes restorative sleep.

Sleep length: Adequate sleep length, typically 7-9 hours each night for adults, improves cognitive function, memory consolidation, immunological function, and hormone regulation. Chronic sleep deprivation, sleep disruptions, or sleep disorders can damage health, cognitive performance, and overall well-being over time.

Avoidance of Harmful Substances

Tobacco and Alcohol: Avoiding tobacco use and excessive alcohol consumption minimizes the risk of chronic diseases, such as lung cancer, cardiovascular disorders, liver diseases, and respiratory conditions. Quitting smoking and reducing alcohol intake contributes to better health outcomes and longevity.

Environmental Toxins: Minimizing exposure to environmental toxins, pollutants, pesticides, and hazardous substances in air, water, and food sources enhances cellular health, detoxification processes, and immune system function. Environmental awareness and lifestyle choices that value clean air, water, and sustainable activities increase general well-being and longevity.

By incorporating these lifestyle elements into everyday activities, individuals can proactively promote their health, enhance longevity, and optimize their chances of aging successfully. Lifestyle choices that focus on nutrition, physical activity, stress management, social connections, sleep quality, and environmental health contribute to a holistic approach to healthy aging and longevity.

CHAPTER 4

SUMMARY AND FUEL FOR A LONGER LIFE

The key to extending life and maximizing health span—the amount of time spent in excellent health free from serious illness or disability—is nutrition. Healthy eating practices coupled with a well-balanced and nutrient-rich diet support immune system performance, cellular health, metabolic resilience, and general well-being as people age.

Plant-Based Priority

Fruits and Vegetables: Including a range of vibrant fruits and vegetables in your daily meals can supply vital vitamins, minerals, antioxidants, and phytonutrients that protect against chronic diseases, maintain cellular health, and reduce inflammation. For a wide variety of nutrients, aim for a rainbow of colors.

Whole Grains: Selecting whole grains delivers more fiber, complex carbs, and micronutrients than refined grains. Examples of whole grains are brown rice, quinoa, oats, and whole wheat products. Whole grains improve cardiovascular health, support healthy digestion, and balance blood sugar levels.

Good Fats

Omega-3 Fatty Acids: Consuming foods high in fatty fish (salmon, mackerel, and sardines), flaxseeds, chia seeds, walnuts, and algae-based supplements promotes cardiovascular health, anti-inflammatory pathways, and brain health. Omega-3 fatty acids improve cognitive performance and lower the chance of age-related cognitive decline.

Monounsaturated Fats: Including foods high in monounsaturated fats, such as avocado, olive oil, almonds, pistachios, and cashews, as well as seeds (sunflower, pumpkin), decreases LDL cholesterol and boosts heart health while supplying vital nutrients and antioxidants.

Trim Proteins

Fish and Poultry: Selecting lean protein sources helps maintain overall nutritional balance, muscular health, and satiety. Examples of these sources are skinless chicken and turkey, fish, shellfish, and plant-based proteins such as lentils, tofu, and tempeh. Omega-3-rich fish provide further cardiovascular benefits.

Limiting Red and Processed Meats: Cutting back on red and processed meats, which are heavy in additives, saturated fats, and sodium, can help reduce the risk of cancer, heart disease, and metabolic disorders linked to overindulgence in meat.

Nutrient-Rich Options

Calcium-Rich Foods: Consuming calcium-rich foods helps maintain bone health and muscle function, and prevents osteoporosis. Examples of these foods include dairy products (low-fat or non-fat alternatives), leafy greens (kale, spinach), fortified plant-based milk, and calcium-fortified meals.

Vitamin D Sources: Getting enough vitamin D improves immune system function, bone health, and mood management. Sources include sunshine exposure, fortified dairy or plant-based milk, fatty fish, and vitamin D supplements (if needed).

Water and Intentional Eating

Water Intake: Maintaining proper hydration levels throughout the day helps with digestion, nutritional absorption, cellular function, and overall hydration levels. Aim for 8 to 10 glasses of water a day, more or less depending on your needs and degree of activity.

Mindful Eating

Mindful eating encourages better food choices, portion control, and digestion. Some of these practices include paying attention to hunger cues, eating carefully, appreciating flavors, and avoiding distractions while eating. Overall nutritional balance and meal satisfaction are supported by mindful eating.

Balance and Diverseness

Portion Control: Mindful eating and portion control techniques encourage fullness, help avoid overindulging, and assist with weight management. Maintaining a healthy weight and lowering the risk of disorders linked to obesity requires striking a balance between energy expenditure and calorie consumption.

Variety and Balance: A well-rounded diet that offers vital nutrients, antioxidants, and phytochemicals is ensured by including a range of foods from various food groups, colors, and textures. Limiting intake of processed foods, sugar, and salt improves general health and lifespan.

Tailored Dietary Plans

Individual Needs: Tailored nutrition regimens that maximize healthspan and foster long-term well-being are made possible by taking into account each person's unique dietary preferences, nutritional needs, food sensitivities, and health objectives. Seeking advice from a qualified dietician or other medical expert might offer tailored direction and assistance.

Long-Term Sustainability: Making dietary adjustments that are pleasurable, long-lasting, and suitable for one's culture encourages people to stick to a healthy diet over time. A positive mindset, realistic goals, and gradual adjustments are key components of a successful long-term diet plan.

In conclusion, the cornerstone for a longer and better life is a balanced and nutrient-rich diet mixed with thoughtful eating practices, hydration, and customized nutrition. Throughout the aging process, cellular health, metabolic resilience, and general well-being are supported by emphasizing plant-based meals, healthy fats, lean meats, nutrient-dense options, moderation, and variety.

PHYSICAL ACTIVITY AND EXERCISE FOR LONGEVITY

Frequent physical activity and exercise are vital elements of a healthy lifestyle that lower the risk of chronic diseases, increase longevity, and enhance quality of life. Including different forms of exercise in daily routines promotes bone density, cognitive function, mental health, physical strength, and cardiovascular health for people of all ages.

Exercise Types

Aerobic Exercise: Activities that increase heart rate, improve cardiovascular fitness, and increase endurance include jogging, cycling, swimming, dancing, and aerobics classes. In addition to lowering the risk of heart disease, stroke, and hypertension, aerobic exercise fortifies the heart, lungs, and circulatory system.

Strength Training: By using weights, resistance bands, or bodyweight exercises, resistance training concentrates on specific muscle groups and enhances their tone, endurance, and strength. Strength training promotes total physical fitness and lifespan by supporting bone health, joint stability, functional mobility, and metabolic rate.

Flexibility and Balance: Stretching exercises, yoga, tai chi, and flexibility exercises improve range of motion, muscular elasticity, and joint flexibility. Exercises for balance enhance postural alignment, stability, and coordination while lowering the risk of falls, accidents, and age-related mobility impairments.

Exercise's Long-Term Benefits

Cardiovascular Health: Regular aerobic exercise decreases blood pressure, improves circulation, strengthens the heart muscle, and lowers cholesterol. Cardiovascular fitness extends life expectancy by lowering the risk of heart disease, stroke, and cardiovascular death.

Musculoskeletal Health: Weight-bearing activities and strength training promote joint health, muscle mass, and bone density. Preserving the strength and functionality of the musculoskeletal system lowers the likelihood of osteoporosis, fractures, arthritis, and age-related mobility problems.

Metabolic Health: By controlling lipid profiles, insulin sensitivity, and blood sugar levels, exercise helps to maintain metabolic health. Long-term metabolic balance is supported by physical activity, which lowers the risk of obesity, metabolic syndrome, type 2 diabetes, and insulin resistance.

Cognitive Function: Memory, mental sharpness, and cognitive function are all improved by regular exercise. Engaging in physical activity lowers the risk of age-related cognitive deficits, Alzheimer's disease, and cognitive decline by stimulating brain-derived neurotrophic factor (BDNF) and promoting neuroplasticity.

Mood and Mental Health: When you exercise, you release endorphins, serotonin, and dopamine—neurotransmitters that lift your spirits, lower stress levels, and promote mental health. Engaging in physical activity can enhance emotional resilience and overall life satisfaction by reducing the incidence of depression, anxiety, and mood disorders.

Recommendations for Exercise

Frequency: Aim for 150 minutes or 75 minutes per week, distributed throughout the week, of moderate-intensity or vigorous-intensity aerobic activity. Include strength training activities for your main muscle groups two to three times a week.

Intensity: Activities like brisk walking, cycling, or dancing that increase breathing and heart rate while allowing for conversation are considered moderate-intensity aerobic exercise. Exercises with a high heart rate and high effort requirements, such as swimming, running, or high-intensity interval training (HIIT), raise the heart rate considerably.

Flexibility and balancing: To increase joint mobility, reduce stiffness, and improve stability, incorporate flexibility exercises, stretching exercises, and balancing activities into your weekly routine.

Progression: To push fitness levels and keep getting health advantages, gradually increase the length, intensity, and complexity of your workouts over time. For individualized exercise advice, speak with a healthcare provider or fitness expert, particularly if you are new to exercising or have any pre-existing medical concerns.

Integrating Exercise into Everyday Life

Active Transportation: For short trips, take the stairs rather than the elevator, walk or ride a bike, and include physical exercise in everyday activities like housework, gardening, or walking meetings.

Group Activities: To stay motivated, mingle, and enjoy physical activity in a supportive setting, join fitness classes, sports clubs, recreational organizations, or community activities.

Technology Tools: To monitor activity levels, set goals, track progress, and get feedback on workouts and daily movement, use fitness trackers, smartphone apps, or wearable devices.

Variety and Enjoyment: To keep yourself interested, avoid boredom, and sustain long-term adherence to exercise regimens, mix in a range of enjoyable physical activities that you enjoy, such as dance, hiking, swimming, yoga, or team sports.

In conclusion, physical activity and exercise are essential for extending life, improving quality of life, and averting chronic illnesses. People can attain optimal physical fitness, mental well-being, and overall health span throughout their lifespan by implementing aerobic exercise, strength training, flexibility, and balancing exercises into their daily lives.

LONGEVITY AND MENTAL HEALTH

Overall well-being and lifespan are greatly impacted by mental health, which also affects the quality of life and physical health outcomes throughout a person's lifetime. Improving psychological well-being, developing emotional resilience, and addressing mental health issues all lead to better results and longer life spans in older populations.

Emotional Hardiness

Coping Skills: Having strong coping mechanisms, such as cognitive restructuring, problem-solving approaches, positive reframing, and stress reduction methods, increases emotional resilience. Resilient people adjust well to hardship, overcome obstacles, and keep their mental health intact when faced with changes and pressures in life.

Emotional Regulation: Mental balance and emotional regulation are supported by self-awareness, emotional intelligence, and mindfulness techniques. Having knowledge of emotions, their causes, and constructive methods to communicate and deal with them promotes stress and psychological resilience.

Social Relations

Social Support Networks: Prolonged mental health and longevity are protected by strong social ties, supportive relationships, and social involvement. Social support networks lessen symptoms of sadness, loneliness, and isolation by offering companionship, emotional support, and a sense of belonging.

Community Involvement: Engaging in volunteer work, social clubs, community service, and group activities helps to create social capital, strengthen interpersonal relationships, and provide a feeling of fulfillment and purpose. Participation in the community improves mental health and increases life satisfaction in general.

Stress Reduction

Stress Reduction Techniques: By using techniques like progressive muscle relaxation, guided imagery, deep breathing exercises, and mindfulness meditation, chronic stress can be lessened in its negative effects on both mental and physical health. Stress management strategies increase resilience to stressors, encourage relaxation, and lessen anxiety.

Work-Life Balance: To promote mental health and avoid burnout, it's important to maintain a healthy work-life balance, set limits, and give self-care, hobbies, and leisure activities a priority. Maintaining a healthy balance between obligations and personal time for leisure, socializing, and relaxation improves longevity.

Mental Wellness

Brain Stimulation: Reading, picking up new skills, solving puzzles, playing games, and pursuing lifelong learning are all examples of intellectually stimulating activities that promote mental agility, memory, and cognitive health. Constant brain stimulation lowers the risk of cognitive decline, protects cognitive function, and encourages neuroplasticity.

Social Interaction: Talking to others, making friends, and taking part in social activities all improve linguistic abilities, social cognition, and cognitive function. As people age, meaningful social connections, conversations, and cooperative activities support mental health and preserve cognitive vibrancy.

Resources and Assistance for Mental Health

Access to Mental Health Services: Having early intervention, symptom management, and recovery from mental health disorders are encouraged by having access to mental health services, counseling, therapy, and psychiatric care as necessary. Mental health practitioners offer evaluation, therapeutic alternatives, and assistance to people dealing with mental health issues.

Educational Resources: Using mental health applications, self-help books, online support groups, and educational resources improve awareness, knowledge, and abilities for successfully managing mental health. Self-care techniques, mindfulness tools, and psychoeducation enable people to actively manage their mental health.

Good Mental Health and Overall Wellness

Gratitude Practices: Developing optimism, gratitude, and a positive view of life improves resilience and psychological well-being. Gratitude exercises, journaling, and emphasizing life's good parts encourage emotional equilibrium, lessen negative thought patterns, and build stress resilience.

Purpose and Meaning: Finding one's values, objectives, and worthwhile pursuits that complement one's sense of purpose enhances psychological health and contentment with life. Longevity and mental health are enhanced by meaningful activities, a positive life narrative, and a sense of purpose in life.

In conclusion, a longer lifespan and a higher quality of life are associated with placing a high priority on mental health, emotional resilience, social relationships, stress management, cognitive stimulation, and overall well-being. Taking care of mental health issues, getting help when needed, and cultivating optimism are all crucial components of a holistic strategy for life expectancy and general well-being.

CULTURAL VIEWS ON LONGEVITY AND AGING

Distinct communities and traditions have very distinct cultural perspectives on aging and longevity, which influence attitudes, beliefs, and actions surrounding aging, eldercare, and the desire for long and healthy lives. To solve age-related issues, encourage intergenerational peace, and promote happy aging experiences, it is imperative to comprehend cultural viewpoints on aging.

Knowledge and Deference to Seniors

Eastern Cultures: Elderly people are valued for their life experience, knowledge, and contributions to the family and community in many Eastern cultures, including China, Japan, and India. Cultural norms that stress intergenerational connections and caregiving responsibilities include filial piety, respect for elders, and multigenerational homes.

Indigenous Cultures: Elders are revered in indigenous societies all over the world as archivists of spiritual advice, oral history, and traditional knowledge. To preserve culture, tell stories, and transmit cultural legacy to future generations, elders are essential.

Social Engagement and Active Aging

Mediterranean Cultures: People from Greece, Italy, and Spain, among other Mediterranean countries, place a high importance on social interactions, active aging, and get-togethers. Mediterranean diet, family meals, regular social interactions, and physical activity are cultural practices linked to lifespan and well-being.

Nordic Cultures: Active lives, outdoor pursuits, and intergenerational social inclusion are valued in Nordic countries, which include those in Denmark, Sweden, and Norway. Nordic aging strategies emphasize chances for lifelong learning and involvement, universal healthcare, and community support.

Cultural Views on the Aging Population

Western Perspectives: In Western societies, youth, productivity, and personal success are highly valued. This can have an impact on attitudes toward retirement and aging, as well as how the general public views older adults. In Western countries, there is constant work to dispel ageist prejudices, create situations that are welcoming to older people, and acknowledge the range of aging experiences.

Global Perspectives: Various cultural perspectives on aging interact in multicultural societies and global communities, offering chances for cross-cultural communication, mutual understanding, and inclusive approaches to aging policies and practices. Respect for cultural variety and common ideals of long life and good health are fostered via cross-cultural interactions and projects.

Longevity Customs and Habits

Blue Zones: These areas of the world, where there is a high concentration of centenarians and long-lived people, provide information about longevity customs and lifestyle choices. Plant-based diets, exercise, meaningful living, robust social networks, and stress-reduction strategies are all prevalent in Blue Zones.

Traditional Chinese Medicine (TCM), Indigenous healing practices, and Indian Ayurveda are examples of traditional healing systems that use holistic approaches to health and well-being that take into account the mental, emotional, physical, and spiritual aspects of aging and longevity.

Relationships Across Generations

Family Dynamics: How aging is viewed and experienced within families is influenced by cultural norms surrounding family structures, caregiving responsibilities, and intergenerational support. Families that value close relationships typically have close-knit networks, multigenerational cohabitation, and shared caregiving obligations.

Community Cohesion: Age-friendly neighborhoods, age-based support networks, and eldercare initiatives encourage older individuals' independence, social inclusion, and quality of life. Culturally sensitive methods of providing housing, healthcare, and aging services take into account the various requirements and preferences that exist in different cultural contexts.

Cultural Storytelling and Imagery

Literature and Arts: Public views of aging, beauty standards, and society's attitudes toward older persons are shaped by cultural narratives, literature, art, and media depictions. Cultural narratives about aging and longevity are shifting in part because of positive portrayals of aging, intergenerational relationships, and elder wisdom.

Educational efforts: To foster understanding, empathy, and respect for a range of aging experiences, cultural backgrounds, and beliefs, educational efforts, awareness campaigns, and cultural competency training programs are implemented. Positive aging environments and age-inclusive communities are fostered via cross-sector collaboration.

To sum up, the way that people and communities tackle issues connected to aging is influenced by the varying values, customs, and social norms that are reflected in the ways that different cultures see aging and longevity. Key ideas for encouraging happy aging experiences and sustaining healthy longevity across cultures include

172 | Page

embracing cultural variety, fostering intergenerational peace, and appreciating the contributions of older persons.

CHAPTER 5

DIVERSITIES IN NATIONAL PERSPECTIVES ON AGEING

Cultural differences in attitudes toward aging are a reflection of the many ideas, values, and social conventions that shape how people view aging, becoming older, and the aging process. Cultural views have an impact on intergenerational connections, aging populations' support from society, and older individuals' well-being by influencing behaviors, expectations, and caring practices.

Honor and Intelligence

Eastern Cultures (such as China and Japan): Aging is seen as a time of wisdom, experience, and spiritual development in many Eastern cultures, which has a strong regard for senior citizens. Elders are frequently seen as sources of wisdom, cultural expertise, and leadership within the family, with intergenerational peace and filial piety serving as fundamental principles.

Indigenous Traditions: Elders are highly valued in indigenous societies all over the world because of their roles as community leaders, storytellers, and keepers of traditions. For their roles in intergenerational mentoring, oral history preservation, and cultural continuity, elders are highly valued.

Family Relationships

Collectivist countries: Families, group decision-making, and intergenerational support are valued highly in cultures that uphold collectivist principles, which include many Asian, African, and Latin American countries. Within networks of extended families, elders are respected and cared for; multigenerational households are not uncommon.

Western Individualism: Western societies place a strong emphasis on personal growth, autonomy, and independence. These ideas can have an impact on how older people are viewed, how they provide care for themselves, and how the community supports them. Sometimes people view aging through the prisms of independence and productivity.

Perspectives on Productivity and Aging

Active Aging: Certain cultures, such as those found in the Nordic and Mediterranean regions, emphasize lifelong learning, social interaction, and active aging as necessary elements of a good aging process. It is recommended that older persons maintain an active lifestyle in terms of their physical, mental, and social well-being.

Retirement and Leisure: Perspectives on retirement, leisure, and work-life balance may differ among cultures.

Retirement can be viewed as a period of leisure, interest, and enjoyment while continuing to give back to the community through mentoring or volunteer work.

Health and Well-Being Views of Health: Preventive care practices, healthcare utilization, and attitudes toward aging-related health issues are all influenced by cultural beliefs about health, sickness, and well-being. Modern healthcare techniques may coexist with herbal treatments, traditional healing methods, and cultural health practices.

Stigma Associated with Mental Health: Help-seeking behaviors, access to mental healthcare, and social support for older persons with mental health issues can be impacted by cultural stigma around mental health conditions, cognitive decline, and emotional well-being.

Cultural Illustrations

Media and Literature: Public attitudes and perceptions of older persons are shaped by cultural narratives, media representations, and literary portrayals of aging. Positive portrayals that emphasize grit, aging well, and leading active lives help to shift cultural perceptions about aging.

Art and Aesthetics: Cultural expressions through aesthetics, art, and customs mirror social ideas of aging gracefully and dignifiedly as well as attitudes toward aging and beauty standards. They also preserve cultural legacy through artistic expression.

Traditions of Longevity

Festivals of Longevity: Several cultures have customs and festivities dedicated to commemorating key life transitions and aging accomplishments, such as centenarian festivals or rites.

Elder hood Ceremonies: Elder hood is associated with a variety of cultural ceremonies, rites of passage, and rituals, all of which have an emphasis on roles, obligations, and social standing.

In conclusion, the diversity of human experiences, values, and customs around the globe is reflected in cultural differences in attitudes toward aging. To create age-inclusive legislation, encourage healthy aging behaviors, and promote intergenerational harmony within varied communities, it is imperative to comprehend and respect cultural viewpoints on aging.

DIFFERENT CULTURES' LONGEVITY CUSTOMS

A vast array of customs, viewpoints, and way of life decisions that are thought to support health, vigor, and a longer life span are included in the category of longevity practices. Different cultural ideas on aging, well-being, and the pursuit of a meaningful life are reflected in these behaviors' variations. Here are a few instances of longevity customs from various cultural backgrounds:

The Blue Zones

The Mediterranean Diet Blue Zone areas include Sardinia (Italy) and Ikaria

(Greece), where a Mediterranean diet high in fruits, vegetables, olive oil, whole grains, and lean proteins is the norm. Longevity, cardiovascular health, and reduced rates of chronic diseases are all linked to this diet.

Physical Activity: Walking, gardening, doing household chores, and leading active lives that enhance muscular strength, cardiovascular health, and general well-being are common forms of regular physical activity in Blue Zones communities.

Social Networks: Blue Zones are known for their robust social networks, intergenerational relationships, and community support, all of which enhance longevity, stress resilience, and emotional well-being.

Chinese Traditional Medicine (TCM)

Herbal Medicine: Traditional Chinese Medicine (TCM) uses herbal medicines, tonics, and nutritional supplements that are meant to enhance longevity, energy, and harmony in the body's Qi (energy) systems.

Qi Gong and acupuncture: These and other related practices, along with Tai Chi, are meant to facilitate better

energy flow, encourage relaxation, and improve general health and vitality.

Nutritional Principles: For maximum health and longevity, Traditional Chinese Medicine (TCM) emphasizes the significance of a balanced diet, moderation in eating, and harmony between the yin and yang qualities of food.

Practices in Okinawa

The Okinawan custom of "Hara Hachi Bu" promotes portion management, digestive health, and a lower caloric intake linked to lifespan. It also encourages eating mindfully and quitting when one is 80% satisfied.

Plant-Based Diet: Okinawans have historically followed a plant-based diet that emphasizes vegetables, beans, tofu, seaweed, and modest amounts of lean meats and fish. This diet has been associated with a decreased risk of chronic illnesses and an enhanced life expectancy.

Active Lifestyle: Okinawans maintain a regular physical activity schedule through walking, gardening, daily routines, and customs that promote cardiovascular health, strength, and mobility.

Native American Traditional Medicine

Herbal Remedies: Indigenous peoples from all over the world have long used plant-based medications, herbal remedies, and other healing techniques to support mental, emotional, and spiritual health.

Ceremonial Practices: Indigenous approaches to health and longevity heavily rely on ceremonies, rituals, and cultural traditions about healing, spirituality, and connection to nature.

Community and Land Connections: Indigenous cultures place a high value on ancestral wisdom, community ties, and holistic approaches to health that take into account mental, emotional, and cultural aspects of well-being.

Dosha Balance in Ayurvedic Medicine: Ayurveda is an age-old Indian medical system that emphasizes balancing the body's doshas (Vata, Pitta, and Kapha) through lifestyle modifications, herbal medicines, and mindfulness exercises.

Yoga and Meditation: Ayurvedic massage treatments, yoga, meditation, and pranayama (breathwork) all help people unwind, reduce tension, and feel more alive overall.

Nutritional Guidelines: Whole foods, seasonal eating, mindful eating, and the significance of gut health, digestion, and nutrient absorption for longevity and overall well-being are all stressed in Ayurvedic dietary guidelines.

In conclusion, varied perspectives on aging, health, and well-being that take into account the mental, emotional,

spiritual, and physical aspects of well-being are reflected in longevity practices across cultural boundaries. These methods frequently place a strong emphasis on social interactions, healthy eating, physical activity, holistic lifestyles, and cultural values that support long life and a feeling of meaning in one's life.

ETHICS AND LONGEVITY

The goal of living longer and improving health span raises difficult moral questions about the rights of the

person, the influence on society, healthcare fairness, and what constitutes a decent life. A variety of viewpoints, moral quandaries, and ethical issues are explored in debates on longevity ethics, which influence our understanding of aging, healthcare, and resource distribution in the context of longer lifespans.

Personal Independence

Right to Choose: The topic of ethical discussions frequently revolves around a person's ability to select

interventions—such as medical procedures, genetic modifications, lifestyle changes, or regenerative therapies—that attempt to lengthen their life expectancy. There are concerns about autonomy, informed consent, and striking a balance between social obligations and personal preferences.

Quality of Life: The quality of life during long life is a topic of discussion in the ethics of longevity. Ethical frameworks emphasize the promotion of healthy, meaningful, and dignified aging experiences that are consistent with personal values and overall well-being, in addition to extended life expectancy.

Equity and Social Justice

Access to Longevity Therapies: Fair access to healthcare services, resources, and therapies that promote longevity for individuals from a variety of socioeconomic backgrounds, marginalized communities, and worldwide populations raises ethical questions. Discussions about longevity ethics must include healthcare equity, affordability, and inequities.

Resource Allocation: The distribution of scarce medical resources in aging societies, the prioritization of healthcare spending, and longevity therapies and regenerative medicine highlight these and other related concerns. Fair distribution, economy, and striking a balance between the requirements of society and individual interests are all highlighted by ethical frameworks.

Extended Durability

Environmental Impact: The effects of population increase, resource use, and longer lifespans on the environment are discussed in discussions of longevity ethics. Extending human life while maintaining the health of the world requires ethical imperatives such as sustainable behaviors, responsible consumerism, and environmental stewardship.

Longer lifespans may have an impact on a variety of economic factors, such as healthcare expenditures, retirement savings, employment participation, and intergenerational financial obligations. The financial viability of social safety nets, pension plans, and healthcare systems in aging nations are topics of ethical debate.

Moral Obligation

Interconnectedness: Individuals, communities, and future generations are all interconnected, according to ethical ideas on longevity. Promoting healthy aging, encouraging social cohesiveness, combating ageism, and developing age-inclusive environments that uphold human rights and dignity throughout life are just a few of the moral obligations.

Ethical Guidelines: Principles like beneficence, non-maleficence, fairness, autonomy, and respect for people are highlighted in ethical frameworks for longevity research, healthcare legislation, and anti-aging interventions. In the quest for greater longevity and health, ethical principles protect human rights and values while assisting in the resolution of difficult moral conundrums.

Perspectives from a Cultural and Spiritual Angle

Cultural Principles: The ethical considerations surrounding aging, longevity, and end-of-life care are influenced by cultural and spiritual beliefs. Inclusive and courteous practices are facilitated by respect for cultural diversity, cultural competency in the healthcare industry, and culturally sensitive approaches to aging and longevity ethics.

Spiritual Well-Being: The human experience of aging, existential meaning, and spiritual well-being may all be discussed in discussions on longevity ethics. Dimensions of spirituality, existential fulfillment, and the pursuit of transcendence and purpose throughout long life are all included in ethical frameworks.

In conclusion, many intricate connections between ethics and longevity call for careful evaluation of people's rights, societal norms, healthcare justice, environmental sustainability, and the moral obligations entailed in prolonging human life. In the quest for longer,

healthier, and more fulfilling lives,
ethical frameworks direct
conversations, laws, and practices that
support human dignity, encourage
ethical decision-making and support
healthy aging.

CHAPTER 6

ETHICAL ASPECTS IN RESEARCH ON LONGEVITY

Understanding the aging process, extending the health span, and promoting longevity are the goals of longevity research. However, it also raises several ethical issues, including those related to individual autonomy, informed consent, equitable access to interventions, societal impacts, and the ethical conduct of scientific research. Longevity research is guided by ethical frameworks that guarantee respect for human rights, moral behavior, and significant contributions to enhancing health and well-being throughout life.

Knowledgeable Consent

Voluntary Participation: To conduct ethical longevity research, participants must voluntarily and knowingly engage in it, guaranteeing that they are aware of the goals, dangers, advantages, and possible consequences of study interventions. Autonomy, respect for human rights, and openness in disclosing the purpose and methods of research are given top priority in informed consent processes.

Vulnerable Populations: Certain groups need special attention, including marginalized communities, older folks, and those with cognitive disabilities. When required, surrogate decision-makers are included, decisional capability evaluations are encouraged, and vulnerable participants are protected by ethical measures.

Benefit-Risk Evaluation

Juggling Risks and Benefits: Research on longevity entails weighing the advantages and disadvantages of various interventions, cures, and preventative measures. Minimizing risks, optimizing potential benefits, and doing risk-benefit analyses that balance participant welfare, safety, and scientific merit are the top priorities when it comes to ethical issues.

Unproven therapies: The use of unproven or possibly dangerous therapies in longevity research is discouraged by ethical norms. Preclinical testing, rigorous scientific evidence, and ethical review procedures are necessary to assess the efficacy and safety of therapies before human trials.

Fairness and Availability

Equitable Recruitment: To ensure generalizability, diversity of perspectives, and equitable access to research opportunities, longevity research should aim for equitable recruitment of different participant communities, especially underrepresented groups.

Healthcare Disparities: Access to healthcare services, healthcare disparities, and the inclusion of people from different socioeconomic backgrounds in research on longevity are all addressed by ethical issues. Fairness, inclusion, and the treatment of health disparities through research projects are all promoted by ethical frameworks.

Confidentiality and Privacy

Data security: Sensitive health information is gathered, stored, and analyzed as part of longevity research. To preserve participant privacy and confidentiality, ethical guidelines place a high priority on data protection, confidentiality, privacy measures, and compliance with data protection laws.

Consent for Data Usage: Longevity research participants must give informed consent for the usage, sharing, and subsequent analysis of their data. Transparency regarding data methods, data security protocols, and participant rights regarding data access and usage are all ethical factors.

Ethical longevity research necessitates the responsible communication of research findings, methodologies, limits, and potential conflicts of interest clearly and factually. Evidence-based decision-making, public trust, and scientific integrity are all enhanced by responsible communication.

Public involvement: To promote awareness of longevity research, ethical concepts, and the societal ramifications of aging-related interventions, ethical concerns also include public involvement, education, and outreach initiatives. Including communities, policymakers, and stakeholders in ethical dialogues encourages responsible research practices and well-informed decision-making.

Long-Term Effects

Long-term societal effects are taken into account by ethical longevity research, and these include healthcare regulations, resource distribution, aging-related societal attitudes, and the moral application of new technologies. Ethical frameworks that support human flourishing, evidence-based policymaking, and beneficial societal effects are all facilitated by responsible research procedures.

Ethical Oversight: Institutional review boards (IRBs), ethics committees, and regulatory agencies oversee research ethics, examine study procedures, and make sure that ethical standards are followed in studies about longevity. Accountability, openness, and the moral conduct of research are encouraged via ethical oversight procedures.

To summarize, participant autonomy, informed consent, benefit-risk assessments, equity and access, privacy protection, responsible communication, and long-term societal repercussions are given top priority when it comes to ethical considerations in longevity research. In addition to protecting human rights and encouraging moral decision-making in the pursuit of expanding scientific knowledge, enhancing health outcomes, and tackling the opportunities and problems associated with an aging population, ethical frameworks also serve as a guide for responsible research conduct.

THE EFFECTS OF EXTENDED LIFESPANS ON SOCIETY

Longer lifespans have significant effects on society in several areas, such as public policy, healthcare, the economy, social structures, and cultural standards. To navigate the opportunities and problems presented by an aging population and to promote inclusive, productive, and healthy societies, these implications must be understood and addressed.

Aging Infrastructure and Healthcare

Systems of Healthcare: Increased demands on healthcare systems due to longer lifespans necessitate improvements in geriatric care, chronic illness management, preventative care, and long-term care services. To meet the health needs of the elderly, encourage healthy aging, and guarantee that they have access to high-quality treatment, the healthcare system must change.

Population Aging: Healthcare systems must effectively manage resources, train medical staff in geriatric care, and adopt age-friendly procedures that improve the quality of life for senior citizens in light of the demographic transition toward an aging population.

Financial Aspects

Pension Systems: Longer life expectancies affect social security, pension funds, and retirement systems.

In aging societies, intergenerational financial support, retirement savings, and sustainable pension schemes become critical.

Workforce Participation: Longer lifespans have an impact on retirement age regulations, workforce dynamics, and chances for older persons to pursue lifetime learning, entrepreneurship, and employment. Workplaces that are age-inclusive, skill development programs, and flexible work schedules encourage economic contributions and healthy aging.

Family dynamics and social structures

Family-Based Caregiving: Living longer may cause a shift in the roles that family members play in providing care, which could have an impact on support networks, intergenerational relationships, and the burden of caregiving. The well-being of caregivers and the independence of older adults are enhanced by policies that support them, respite care services, and community-based care options.

Living arrangements: To accommodate an older population, changes must be made to housing options, living arrangements, and community infrastructure. Independent living, social inclusion, and active aging are encouraged by age-friendly housing, accessible settings, and caring communities.

Cultural Transitions and Perceptions of Aging Ageism: The social inclusion, opportunities, and perceptions of older persons are influenced by societal attitudes regarding aging, ageism, and stereotypes. Age-friendly societies are those that support good aging narratives, challenge ageist prejudices, and promote intergenerational understanding.

Cultural norms: How societies view and sustain an aging population is shaped by cultural values, traditions, and interactions between generations. In aging societies, cultural diversity and well-being are fostered by inclusive practices, culturally sensitive approaches, and appreciation for the variety of aging experiences.

Governance and Policy

Age-Friendly Policies: Developing healthcare reforms, social protection programs, and community services that cater to the requirements of the aging population is a major responsibility of governments, legislators, and advocacy groups. The intricate problems associated with longer lifespans are addressed by multisectoral methods, stakeholder participation, and evidence-based policymaking.

Extended-Term Scheduling: Well-being across the lifetime is supported by long-term planning, deliberate investments in aging research, public health campaigns, and infrastructure development. Sustainable solutions for an aging society are facilitated by collaborative efforts, data-driven decision-making, and anticipatory governance.

In conclusion, longer lifespans have significant societal ramifications that call for proactive measures, cross-sector collaboration, and creative problem-solving. To create vibrant societies that take advantage of the potential that comes with longevity while also effectively addressing its issues, we must promote healthy aging, age-friendly surroundings, social inclusion, economic opportunity, and equal access to resources.

JUGGLING LIFE EXPECTANCY AND QUALITY OF LIFE

Making sure that an extended lifetime is accompanied by a high standard of physical health, mental well-being, social relationships, and general life satisfaction is necessary to strike a balance between longevity and quality of life. While living longer is undoubtedly a major accomplishment, preserving a high standard of living as one age is just as crucial. The following are important factors and methods for striking this balance:

Difference between Lifespan and Health span: The term "health span" describes the length of time a person spends in good health, devoid of serious illnesses or disabilities. Prioritizing both lifespan and health span is necessary to strike a balance between longevity and quality of life, ensuring that people not only live longer but also continue to enjoy optimal health and well-being.

Preventive Healthcare: By lowering the burden of chronic diseases, controlling risk factors, and improving general well-being, a focus on preventive healthcare, routine screenings, healthy lifestyle choices, and early intervention techniques increase health span.

Wholesome Wellness Physical Well-Being: Maintaining physical health and energy throughout life requires promoting physical exercise, a healthy diet, enough sleep, frequent checkups with the doctor, and access to healthcare services.

Mental Health: Improving emotional resilience, addressing mental health issues, offering mental health support services, and encouraging constructive coping mechanisms all enhance mental health and quality of life.

Social Links: Emotional support, company, and a sense of belonging— all of which improve quality of life— come from sustaining social links, meaningful relationships, social engagement, and community involvement.

Personal Preferences and Objectives

Human-Centered Healthcare: Finding a balance between longevity and quality of life requires an understanding of personal preferences, values, aspirations, and objectives in life. Person-centered care approaches customize lifestyle advice, support services, and medical interventions to fit each patient's unique needs and preferences.

Planning for Care: People can make educated decisions about their care and quality of life when advance care planning is discussed, healthcare preferences are made clear, end-of-life wishes are recorded, and individual autonomy is respected.

Adopting a Healthier Lifestyle

Exercise and Diet: Healthy lifestyle practices, strength training, flexibility exercises, balanced diets, and regular physical activity all contribute to an individual's increased physical fitness, mobility, and general well-being as they age.

Stress Management: By teaching people how to reduce stress, and anxiety, and foster mental resilience for a higher quality of life, people can also learn mindfulness exercises, relaxation techniques, and coping skills.

Community Involvement and Social Support

Social Networks: Developing friendships, familial ties, and social support systems improves overall life satisfaction, increases emotional resilience, and lessens feelings of loneliness.

Community Involvement: Engaging in volunteer work, social clubs, and group activities contributes to a higher quality of life by fostering a sense of purpose, social involvement, and fulfillment.

Palliative and terminal illness care

Palliative Care: Enhancing quality of life, fostering comfort, and respecting individual dignity and choices are all achieved by combining palliative care services with pain management, symptom relief, and holistic support for those with serious illnesses or old age.

End-of-Life Organization: To ensure that people receive care that is in line with their beliefs and wishes and improves the quality of life at the end of life, it is important to have open discussions regarding end-of-life care preferences, advance directives, hospice care options, and spiritual or cultural considerations.

In conclusion, achieving a balance between longevity and quality of life necessitates a comprehensive strategy that emphasizes social relationships, mental and physical health, individual preferences, healthy lifestyle choices, social support, and individualized care for the duration of one's life. People can live longer, better, and more meaningful lives while still retaining a high quality of life by focusing on both lifespan and health span.

CHAPTER 7

OPPORTUNITIES FOR RADICAL LIFE ADDITION

The possible benefits and ramifications of greatly extending human lifetime beyond existing bounds are examined in this chapter. Here's a summary of the subject:

Current Longevity Trends

Medical Advancements: Extensive advancements in biotechnology, regenerative medicine, anti-aging medicines, and medical research have resulted in improved health outcomes and longer life expectancies for numerous age-related ailments.

Initiatives for Healthy Aging: Disease prevention, well-being, and healthy aging have been made possible in part by public health initiatives, lifestyle modifications, preventative healthcare, and awareness campaigns.

New Research Areas and Technologies

Engineering Genetics: Targeting genetic variables linked to aging, and diseases, and improving life expectancy may be possible with the help of genetic engineering, gene editing methods (such as CRISPR-Cas9), and personalized medicine.

Regenerative medicine aims to repair age-related damage, restore tissue function, and increase longevity through the use of stem cell therapies, tissue engineering, organ regeneration, and cellular rejuvenation techniques.

Anti-Aging Interventions: A variety of cutting-edge medications, senolytics, mitochondrial rejuvenation, epigenetic alterations, and mimicking caloric restriction is being studied as possible anti-aging treatments that may prolong life and enhance health outcomes.

Considerations for Society and Ethics

Ethical Debates: Radical life extension discussions bring up ethical issues related to equity, access to life-extending technology, healthcare priorities, resource allocation, environmental effects, and the long-term effects on people's well-being and society.

Quality of Life: To guarantee that an extended lifespan is accompanied by excellent health, happiness, fulfilling experiences, and social ties, it is crucial to strike a balance between longevity and quality of life factors.

Consequences for the Economy and Society

Workforce and Retirement: To account for longer lifespans and aging populations, laws governing retirement ages, labor force participation, pension plans, and economic planning may need to be adjusted as a result of increased life expectancy.

Healthcare Systems: As people live longer, there are possibilities and difficulties for the healthcare system, including aging infrastructure, long-term care services, workforce development, and sustainable finance options.

Effects on Society Over Time

Cultural Shifts: Extending life beyond reason may result in changes in how people view aging, life stages, family dynamics, job paths, societal roles, and expectations for various stages of life.

Interdisciplinary Collaboration: To effectively address the complex prospects and problems of radical life extension, collaboration between scientists, ethicists, policymakers, healthcare practitioners, economics, social scientists, and stakeholders is essential.

Possible Advantages and Difficulties

Benefits: Radical life extension may lead to improved productivity, a longer lifetime, a lower rate of illness, scientific discoveries, the sharing of information between generations, and chances for personal development and fulfillment.

Difficulties: Difficulties may include unequal access to healthcare, unethical decisions, existential concerns, environmental effects, social cohesiveness, intergenerational equity, and the need to rethink social norms and institutions in light of longer lifespans.

To sum up, the potential for drastic life extension raises fascinating scientific questions, moral dilemmas, and societal ramifications. To successfully navigate the challenges of greatly extending the human lifespan, careful investigation, interdisciplinary cooperation, open communication, and responsible decision-making are needed. To shape a future in which longer lifespans foster well-being, innovation, and thriving societies, the quest for longevity must be balanced with considerations of quality of life, equity, sustainability, and ethical standards.

THE SOCIAL AND ETHICAL DIFFICULTIES OF EXTREME LONGEVITY

We explore the intricate problems and factors to be taken into account when greatly extending human lifespans becomes possible. An examination of the main difficulties in this field is provided here:

Distribution of Resources

Healthcare Prioritization: Given the heightened healthcare requirements of an aging society, exceptionally long lifespans may prompt inquiries regarding the distribution of healthcare resources. Prioritizing life-extending therapies over pressing medical demands or public health concerns might provide ethical conundrums.

Economic Impact: Longer life expectancies have an impact on social security, pension plans, healthcare costs, and labor relations. As a result, long-term planning, sustainable economic models, and fair resource allocation among generations are necessary.

Access to Life-Extending Technologies and Social Equity: If life-extending treatments or technologies become primarily accessible to affluent populations, there may be worries about social inequality and access discrepancies, which could lead to growing health disparities and moral dilemmas with fairness and social justice.

Longevity Divide: There may be a "longevity divide" in which people who have access to therapies that extend life enjoy longer periods of health and well-being while underprivileged populations endure lower life expectancies, health inequalities, and obstacles to receiving healthcare.

Existential and Moral Issues to Be Considered

Meaning of Life: Philosophical inquiries regarding the meaning and purpose of life, individual identity, existential fulfillment, and the significance of human experiences during prolonged lifespans may arise from very long lifespans.

Quality of Life: Preserving a high quality of life is central to ethical discourse, as it guarantees that an increased life expectancy is concomitant with optimal health, happiness, dignity, autonomy, meaningful connections, and chances for individual development and accomplishment.

Social Organization and Dynamics

Intergenerational Dynamics: As people live longer, there may be changes in family structures, caregiving duties, societal roles, and intergenerational relationships. These changes can affect support networks, social cohesion, and family dynamics.

Cultural Norms: Cultural sensitivity, age-friendly practices, and inclusive approaches to aging are necessary because societal attitudes regarding aging, ageism, and stereotypes may affect perceptions, expectations, and society's responses to extreme longevity.

Making Ethical Decisions and Policies

Ethical Frameworks: Addressing the ethical issues of extreme longevity and guaranteeing respect for human rights, dignity, autonomy, and well-being in healthcare, research, and policy development requires the development of ethical frameworks, guidelines, and decision-making processes.

Policy Implications: Creating rules that strike a balance between the goal of longevity and social effect, equity, resource allocation, informed consent, privacy protection, end-of-life care, and societal values is a difficult task for legislators.

Sustainability of the Environment

Population Growth: Living longer may have an impact on ecological footprints, resource consumption, environmental sustainability, and the long-term survival of ecosystems and natural resources.

Green Longevity: Ideas like "green longevity" highlight the need for eco-friendly living, conscientious consumption, and environmental stewardship in fostering aging societies that are both healthy and sustainable.

In conclusion, navigating the complications of greatly extending the human lifespan requires careful analysis, interdisciplinary collaboration, public discourse, and ethical decision-making. These are the ethical and social problems associated with extreme longevity. To shape a future where longer lifespans positively contribute to human happiness and well-being, it is imperative to strike a balance between the quest for longevity and ethical values, equity, social effect, quality of life, cultural diversity, and environmental sustainability.

LIFESPAN IN SCIENCE FICTION AND FUTURE SCENARIOS

We investigate the representation, imagining, and exploration of the idea of a longer human lifespan in literature and science fiction. This is an examination of this intriguing subject:

Concepts and Illustrations

Science fiction frequently depicts circumstances in which characters acquire near-immortality or immortality as a result of cutting-edge medical advancements, genetic modifications, or advanced technologies. These stories examine the ramifications, moral conundrums, and philosophical issues raised by eternal life.

Anti-aging technology: Regenerative medicine, life-extending therapies, and anti-aging technology that dramatically lengthen human lifespans are commonplace in science fiction. These stories explore the ethical dilemmas, personal decisions, and societal effects of excessive longevity.

Social and Moral Consequences

Social Structures: Science fiction delves into how longer life spans affect cultural conventions, family dynamics, labor force participation, retirement ideas, and relationships between generations. Speculative futures frequently show age-diverse communities and the potential and problems they bring.

Ethical Dilemmas: About radical life extension, fictional stories address ethical questions about resource allocation, access to life-extending technologies, social equality, existential boredom, purposelessness, and the meaning of existence in a post-death society.

Technological Progress

Genetic Engineering: In science fiction, aging processes, cellular damage, and biological immortality are all possible for humans through genetic engineering, gene editing, and customized medication.

The concepts of mind-uploading, digital consciousness, transhumanism, and the possibility of transferring human consciousness onto artificial or virtual substrates, overcoming biological constraints, and obtaining endless lifespans are all explored in speculative futures.

Effects on Culture and Psychology

Cultural Shifts: Fictional accounts show how attitudes about aging, cultural values, societal expectations, ideas of success and achievement, and the quest for meaningful experiences across extended lifespans are all altered by prolonged life.

Psychological Difficulties: Science fiction explores the psychological difficulties of living forever, such as existential crises, identity loss, connections with others, dealing with the past, and discovering meaning and fulfillment in an endless life.

Visions of the Dystopian and Utopian

Utopian Visions: Some theories of the future offer utopian pictures of prolonged lifespans in which society prospers, defeats age-related illnesses, establishes social harmony, and seizes the chance to live forever and advance both individually and as a whole.

On the other hand, dystopian scenarios including prolonged lifespans that result in societal stratification, elitism, inequality, authoritarian control, existential ennui, loss of humanity, and unanticipated repercussions of immortality are frequently explored in science fiction.

Thoughts on the Nature of Humans

Fictional stories invite contemplation on the connections between identity, human experience, mortality, and the fleeting nature of relationships, life's milestones, and personal development.

Speculative futures warn against hubris, excessive dependence on technology, the quest for immortality at all costs, and the unexpected repercussions of tampering with life and death.

In summary, the concept of longevity in science fiction and speculative futures provides a framework for

examining existential issues, moral conundrums, cultural changes, technology advancements, and the human condition in a world where the lines separating life and death are blurred. These stories encourage introspection, creativity, and critical discussion about the advantages and disadvantages of greatly expanding the human lifespan.

CONCLUSION

SUMMARY OF SIGNIFICANT DISCOVERIES AND PERCEPTIONS

Imagining Immortality: Science fiction typically tackles the subject of immortality or near-immortality gained through sophisticated technologies, genetic upgrades, or futuristic medical advances. These scenarios prompt inquiries into the outcomes, moral quandaries, and philosophical obstacles linked to immortality.

Anti-Aging Technologies: Fictional narratives typically feature anti-aging technologies, regenerative medicine, and life-extending procedures that dramatically enhance human longevity. These stories explore the effects on society, individual decision-making, and ethical dilemmas related to excessive longevity.

Societal and Ethical Implications: Science fiction storylines explore the effects of longer lifespans on societal structures, cultural norms, family dynamics, workforce engagement, retirement notions, and intergenerational relationships. Additionally, these advancements give rise to ethical quandaries concerning the distribution of resources, availability of life-prolonging technology, fairness in society, and the existential significance of existence in a world where mortality is no longer unavoidable.

Technological Advancements

Speculative futures anticipate progress in genetic engineering, gene editing, personalized medicine, mind-uploading, and transhumanism that empower people to manipulate aging processes, restore cellular damage, and attain biological immortality. These technological capabilities spark discussions about the bounds of human potential and the risks and rewards of pushing those boundaries.

Cultural and Psychological Impact

Fictional narratives explore how longer lifespans affect cultural values, attitudes about aging, societal expectations, concepts of success and achievement, and the quest for meaningful experiences across extended lifespans. In addition, they explore the psychological difficulties associated with living endlessly, such as existential crises, loss of identity, connections with mortal others, and the search for meaning in an everlasting existence.

Speculative futures offer both utopian and dismal perspectives on the idea of living longer lives. Some tales portray a world in which mankind flourishes, attains social harmony, and embraces the possibilities of living indefinitely. However, other narratives warn about the dangers of societal divisions, inequality, authoritarian rule, the erosion of human qualities, and the unforeseen negative effects of immortality.

Contemplations on Human Nature

These stories stimulate contemplations on death, individuality, the human condition, and the temporary nature of life's significant events, accomplishments, relationships, and personal development. They also caution against arrogance, overreliance on technology, and the goal of immortality without addressing the ethical, cultural, and psychological ramifications.

In summary, "Longevity in Science Fiction and Speculative Futures" offers as a thought-provoking investigation of human needs, concerns, aspirations, and ethical considerations in picturing a society where the bounds of life and death are redefined. These narratives give unique insights into the human condition, technical potentials, societal transformations, and the complexities of extending the human lifetime dramatically.

LOOKING AHEAD: THE EVOLVING LANDSCAPE OF LONGEVITY

It covers the future trends, difficulties, possibilities, and breakthroughs impacting the subject of longevity. Here's a summary of what to expect in the growing landscape of longevity:

Advancements in Biotechnology and Medicine

Breakthroughs in genetic engineering, regenerative medicine, and individualized treatments are likely to change longevity research.

Emerging technologies such as CRISPR-Cas9, gene editing, and precision medicine hold promise for tackling age-related disorders and prolonging health span.

Anti-Aging Therapies and Interventions

Continued research and development in anti-aging medications, senolytics, stem cell treatments, and rejuvenation tactics attempt to slow down or reverse the aging process.

Clinical trials and advances in longevity-enhancing therapies give hope for improving health outcomes and quality of life in older persons.

Digital Health and Wearable Technology

The integration of digital health tools, wearables, health monitoring devices, and AI-driven diagnostics will empower consumers to manage their health, track biomarkers, and make informed decisions about lifestyle and healthcare choices.

Telemedicine, remote monitoring, and virtual care platforms will expand access to healthcare services and promote preventive care activities.

Longevity and Environmental Sustainability

Sustainable aging initiatives, eco-friendly behaviors, green longevity principles, and health-promoting surroundings will focus on planetary health, environmental sustainability, and healthy aging.

Addressing environmental issues, pollution, climate change consequences, and lifestyle choices will be crucial to improving lifespan and well-being.

Precision Aging and Personalized Health

Advances in precision aging, biomarkers of aging, epigenetics, and omics technology will enable personalized health assessments, tailored therapies, and unique aging trajectories.

Tailored lifestyle suggestions, nutritional treatments, and wellness regimens based on genetic, metabolic, and physiological profiles will maximize health span and resilience.

Ethical and Social Considerations

Ethical frameworks, regulatory norms, and policy discussions will address the ethical issues of radical life extension, genetic enhancements, and access to life-extending technologies.

Social fairness, healthcare inequities, cultural diversity, informed consent, privacy protection, and end-of-life care will remain significant areas of concern in the shifting landscape of longevity.

Collaborative Research and Interdisciplinary Approaches

Collaborative efforts among scientists, healthcare professionals, policymakers, ethicists, technologists, and stakeholders will drive advances in longevity research, innovation, and implementation.

Interdisciplinary approaches, data-sharing efforts, worldwide alliances, and knowledge exchange platforms will expedite breakthroughs in the field of longevity.

Public Awareness and Education

Public awareness campaigns, education programs, and science communication activities will enhance understanding, engagement, and informed decision-making on longevity, healthy aging, and preventative healthcare.

Addressing myths, stigma, and ageist attitudes will develop age-friendly communities, inclusivity, and good views toward aging.

In conclusion, the emerging landscape of longevity provides great potential for extending health span, improving quality of life, and resolving age-related difficulties through scientific discoveries, technology innovations, ethical concerns, and collaborative activities. Looking ahead, a holistic strategy that blends scientific research, digital health solutions, environmental sustainability, customized medicine, and social equality will define a future where people live longer, healthier, and more satisfying lives.